EXCITING DISCOVERIES

The health maverick in each of us—the one that governs those unique needs which do not conform to "normal" standards—can now be satisfied through this newly explored family of food "accessories." With lecithin, if you can't make enough yourself, to conquer cholesterol and aid memory; or inositol, which helps the liver manage fat and helps nerves grow. These nutrients which possess powerful therapeutic value for specific individuals occupy one of the most exciting new areas in nutritional development.

ABOUT THE AUTHOR AND EDITORS

Jeffrey Bland, Ph.D., is a promoter of good health — whether he is teaching, practicing, lecturing or writing, he is actively committed to the idea that the relationship between health and lifestyle when properly revised leads to longer, healthier lives and more productive contributions to the survival of our species. A Ph.D. in biochemistry, he is Professor of Nutritional Biochemistry at the University of Puget Sound, Director of the Bellevue Redmond Medical Laboratory and the dedicated advocate of healthful common sense from the lecture platform primarily to physicians, dentists and other scientists. His latest book is *Your Health Under Siege* and he has also authored many magazine articles.

Richard A. Passwater, Ph.D., is one of the most called-upon authorities for information relating to preventive health care. A noted biochemist, he is credited with popularizing the term "supernutrition" largely as a result of having written two bestsellers on the subject — *Supernutrition: Megavitamin Revolution* and *Supernutrition for Healthy Hearts.* His other books include *Easy No-Flab Diet, Cancer and Its Nutritional Therapies,* and the recently published *Selenium as Food & Medicine.* He has just completed a new book on *Hair Analysis* with Elmer M. Cranton, M.D.

Earl Mindell, R.Ph., Ph.D., combines the expertise and working experience of a pharmacist with extensive knowledge in most of the nutrition areas. His book *Earl Mindell's Vitamin Bible* is now a million-copy bestseller; and his more recent *Vitamin Bible for Your Kids* may very well duplicate his first *Bible's* publishing history. Dr. Mindell's popular *Quick & Easy Guide to Better Health* was just published by Keats Publishing.

Volume 1

CHOLINE, LECITHIN, INOSITOL AND OTHER "ACCESSORY" NUTRIENTS

THE EXCITING NEW USES OF POWERFUL NUTRIENTS FOR PEOPLE WITH SPECIAL NEEDS

by Jeffrey Bland, Ph.D.

Keats Publishing, Inc. New Canaan, Connecticut

Choline, Lecithin, Inositol and Other "Accessory" Nutrients is not intended as medical advice. Its intention is solely informational and educational. Please consult a medical or health professional should the need for one be warranted.

Contents

I INTRODUCING THE ACCESSORY NUTRIENTS IN HEALTH PROMOTION

The role that vitamins and minerals play in human nutrition has been established through years of clinical and biochemical research. Their important function in activating specific enzymes and serving as cellular protective agents is now accepted, and the therapeutic usefulness of vitamin and mineral factors when given in doses above that of the Recommended Dietary Allowances is receiving greater and greater attention.

There is another class of nutrients which are concentrated from food and are now receiving equal attention. These are not members of the essential nutrient family, but rather are termed "accessory food factors." To distinguish between an accessory food factor and an essential vitamin or mineral it is important to recognize their differences.

An essential nutrient is a substance, such as vitamin B1 (thiamine) or vitamin B2 (riboflavin), or vitamin C (ascorbic acid), which cannot be manufactured within the human body and must be gotten from the diet where another plant or animal has produced it. It must be consumed in the human diet in adequate amounts to meet the needs of health promotion.

There are a few essential nutrients that actually fall outside this rigorous definition and still are considered to be vitamin factors. An example is vitamin D, which can be manufactured in a person's body by exposure to full-spectrum sunlight, or vitamin B12 which can be partially manufactured by bacteria in the gastrointestinal tract, or vitamin B3 (niacin) which can be partly manufactured in the liver from dietary tryptophan, although not at levels adequate to meet the needs of most healthy people.

We still consider these agents to be vitamin factors since their ability to be manufactured in the human body is inadequate for prevention of known vitamin deficiency diseases, such as pernicious anemia with vitamin B12 or pellagra with vitamin B3, and therefore must be gotten from the diet.

The accessory food factors, on the other hand, are materials which are manufactured within the human body, at levels which for most individuals would be considered "adequate." The important distinction is that many of these accessory metabolites native to the human body may not be manufactured at *optimal* levels for the promotion of health, and therefore may be more useful when taken in the diet or as a food supplement. This frames the basic concept of the therapeutic use of accessory food factors in clinical nutrition. Any person may require one or more of these accessory food factors to be consumed in greater amounts than the average diet provides because of his or her unique health or genetic state.

This new list of nutrients which may possess powerful therapeutic value when given in enhanced doses to specific individuals is one of the most exciting new areas of clinical nutrition. A partial list of such factors is shown below:

Representative Accessory Nutrients
Choline (lecithin)
Inositol
Taurine
Carnitine
Octacosanol
Dimethylglycine
Specific amino acids
Vegetable gums
Garlic concentrate
Saponins
Dietary fibers
Bioflavonoids

Xanthopylls
Beta-carotene
Specific oil concentrates (i.e., marine lipids such as EPA)

To illustrate the principle of the use of a therapeutic food factor in clinical nutrition one need only look at a condition such as phenylketonuria. Phenylketonuria is a genetic condition in which an infant is born with the inability to metabolize the amino acid phenylalanine properly in the diet. This amino acid comes from dietary protein. When it cannot be properly metabolized, it builds up in the body and supposedly produces mental retardation.

Traditionally, the treatment of this condition has been to put the infant on a low phenylalanine diet. Recently, however, investigators have suggested that phenylketonuria may be better treated by administering augmented supplies of the amino acid tyrosine, made from phenylalanine, which may be deficient due to a metabolic block. In clinical studies when tyrosine was administered to infants who had phenylketonuria in the absence of a phenylalanine restricted diet, their IQ and performance actually were better than when the infants had been placed on a phenylalanine restricted diet.[1] This indicates that possibly for these individuals the symptoms of retardation are really a result of tyrosine deficiency, and for them tyrosine becomes an essential amino acid that must be acquired through diet or supplements. In such a case an accessory food factor becomes an essential nutrient in some individuals. This is called the justification hypothesis, which suggests that certain nutrients usually manufactured in the individual's own body may be essential in certain individuals because of their genetic limitation in the ability to manufacture the substance in adequate quantities.[2]

The proposal of Dr. Roger Williams some forty years ago of biochemical individuality is the theme upon which this particular concept is based. Dr. Williams talks about genetotrophic diseases being diseases which can be ameliorated or prevented when an augmented supply of one or more constituents within food are supplied, based upon the individual's genetic uniqueness.[3]

Specific health or medical conditions may also require an enhanced intake of one of the accessory food factor family. The recognition of specific biochemical needs for these accessory food factors has opened the door for a whole new field of clinical nutrition.

This monograph will discuss the clinical usefulness of four such accessory food factors which represent the general field. The future for the use of these substances is very rich, and as we learn more about food concentrates and the principles within them, we begin to recognize the panoramic clinical utility of the accessory food factors.

Recently, such essential oils as evening primrose oil and fish oil from cold water fish (such as mackerel and salmon) providing Omega 3 EPA have shown usefulness in enhancing the immune function and reducing blood cholesterol and the risk of heart disease.[4,5] These are two additional examples of accessory food factors which have been demonstrated to have therapeutic benefit in controlled human studies.

The following volume frames the discussion of the accessory food factors—choline, lecithin, inositol and beta-carotene. Volume II of this series will go on to discuss additional accessory food factors—taurine, carnitine, octacosanol and glucomannan.

II CHOLINE AND LECITHIN

DIETARY SOURCES AND THE DIFFERENCE BETWEEN CHOLINE AND LECITHIN

Choline is a well recognized member of the B complex vitamin family; however, dietary deficiency of choline has only been demonstrated to produce liver problems in animals, and no acute deficiency has been seen in humans. This is in part a result of the fact that choline can be manufactured in the human body and therefore is not truly an essential nutrient, but rather a member of the accessory food factor family.[6]

Choline has been used therapeutically in human studies to prevent alcoholic cirrhosis and liver damage, but with varying success.[7] In the body, choline is utilized as a substance from which phosphatidylcholine, which is called lecithin, is manufactured. As seen in Figure 1, lecithin is made up of a glycerol backbone with two fatty acids and a phosphatidylcholine residue combined chemically. In the lecithin molecule the fatty acids can either be of the saturated or unsaturated fatty acid families. The more highly saturated lecithins coming from animal sources are solid at room temperature, whereas the more unsaturated lecithins are generally from vegetable origin and are liquid at room temperature. The body manufactures lecithin in the liver, which it utilizes for the formation of proper bile.

This lecithin is manufactured from choline that comes from both the diet and the body's own manufacturing process.

The concentration of choline in the body and the blood depends upon dietary choline intake. Dietary lecithin will also elevate tissue and serum choline levels; foods such as eggs, liver, soybeans and peanuts are the highest dietary sources. Once the dietary lecithin has been taken in, it is broken down in the intestinal tract to substances which are absorbed into the blood and then remade into lecithin in the liver. A food-ingested dose of choline at the level of 0.3 grams per kilogram of body weight will increase the blood level of choline by 400 percent, and this will last for twelve hours.[8] The normal dietary intake of choline is approximately 300 mg a day, coming from a wide variety of foods. Lecithin has been utilized as a dietary source of choline for certain therapeutic trials, but it should be recalled that commercial lecithin has a wide variety of compositions, as it relates to their choline content. The highly concentrated and purified lecithins, in which the composition is greater than 30 percent phosphatidylcholine, will supply the highest amounts of choline and lead to the greatest blood elevations of choline after oral administration.

USE OF LECITHIN IN HUMAN BIOCHEMISTRY

Choline and lecithin are absorbed in the upper intestine and seem to be transmitted to the blood by what is known as passive diffusion, meaning the higher the amount in the diet, the more will appear in the blood. One of the major problems in utilizing choline in large doses as a supplement is that part of it is broken down in the intestines to a substance called trimethylamine, which has the odor of rotten fish associated with it. The intestinal bacteria manufacture trimethylamine from high levels of dietary choline and the individual takes on a characteristic odor as a result of the choline therapy. It has been found that the use of lecithin in high levels will deliver to the blood high levels of choline, but will not be cleaved in the intestinal tract to trimethylamine, and so will avoid the unpleasant fishy odor.

There are a number of tissues which have been shown to utilize the high blood levels of choline in the manufacture of specific substances such as lecithin or acetylcholine within them. (Acetylcholine is secreted at the nerve junction which helps transport messages across the nerve junctions, so that proper nervous system function can result. It is a well-known member of the neurotransmitter family.) The tissues which use choline include the brain, kidney, liver and spleen. Three tissues are known to be able to synthesize choline, and this is why it is not generally considered an essential nutrient. Those tissues in the human are the liver, the testes and the heart. However, these three organs are capable of making only about 15 percent of the daily need, and therefore if the diet does not contain adequate levels of choline or lecithin, then subtle signs of undernutrition can appear. The major role of choline, once absorbed in the body and transported in the blood to the tissues that need it, is as a stimulator of the synthesis of lecithin as a raw material from which acetylcholine is synthesized. Choline also functions as a member of the lipotrophic vitamin family involved in methyl donation for the conversion to another member of this lipotrophic family, betaine.

The therapeutic usefulness of lecithin and choline is to a great extent related to their readiness to be converted to acetylcholine.

CHOLINE IN FETAL DEVELOPMENT AND THE NEWBORN

It has been found that newborns have extremely high choline content in their blood, which seems to be necessary for the manufacture of the nervous system insulator called myelin, and for the synthesis of the membranes of many cells within the nervous system and brain.[10] Deficiencies of choline in the newborn or the fetus may produce profound developmental abnormalities as it relates to the nervous system. Human milk, which is 3.8 percent fat, as compared to cow's milk, which is 3 to 5 percent fat, has much higher levels of lecithin than cow's milk. These lecithins are used by the developing fetus for the manufacture of a lung surfactant material which prevents infection and other lung disorders once the fetus has been delivered. Inappropriately low manufacture of this lung surfactant material can lead to respiratory distress in the infant, one of the major neonatal problems, particularly in premature birth. Proper transport of choline across the placental barrier from the mother's diet seems very important in establishing optimal choline levels for the developing fetus. Also, mother's milk, being higher in lecithin than cow's milk, may be extremely important in providing optimal levels of choline for the developing nervous system of the infant.[11]

THERAPEUTIC BENEFITS OF CHOLINE/LECITHIN ADMINISTRATION

Choline has been used to treat certain neurological diseases for over fifty years when given therapeutically. The major sites of action when choline is given therapeutically are the nervous system, the cardiovascular system and the liver. In the nervous system choline has been found to stimulate the production of acetylcholine in the brain which is used as a neurotransmitter involved in arousal, learning, REM sleep and motor activity.[12]

Therapeutically, it has been used in doses of about 9 to 12 grams of choline chloride per day to treat tardive dyskinesia, a neurological condition produced as a side effect of the use of anti-schizophrenic medication. Tardive dyskinesia results when there is inadequate manufacture of acetylcholine in certain neurons in the brain, and enhanced levels of dietary choline or lecithin will normalize this synthesis and remove the symptoms of fine motor shaking, slurred speech and palsy-like reactions of the nervous system. All known neuroleptic drugs have the side effect of tardive dyskinesia associated with them, and these appear in approximately 50 percent of the patients treated with these medications. At this time the only effective treatment for tardive dyskinesia is the administration of therapeutic doses of oral choline or lecithin, with lecithin apparently preferable to choline.[13]

Other motor problems such as Huntington's disease and Gilles de la Tourette syndrome have also been suggested to be responsive to enhanced dietary choline or lecithin.

Recently, one of the clinical applications of enhanced lecithin and choline consumption has been improved memory in the presenile demented patient. Memory loss in these patients seems to be a result of the loss of acetylcholine in the septo-hypocampal cholinergic neuron in the brain, and enhanced dietary levels of lecithin or choline will override this difficulty.[14]

It is well known that even healthy humans who are treated with anticholinergic drugs may develop memory loss; the use of dietary supplements of lecithin or choline can reduce the symptoms.

Alzheimer's disease is a condition associated with memory loss in the aged individual and has been suggested to be related to excessive aluminum exposure and concentration of aluminum in the brain. Recently, lecithin has been found helpful in the Alzheimer's disease patient.

One of the most exciting new developments in the use of lecithin therapeutically is the management of manic depression, along with lithium. Lithium improves the uptake of choline across the blood/brain barrier, and the administration of lecithin along with lithium will reduce the need for lithium considerably, thereby improving the levels of acetylcholine. Seventy-five percent of patients in a clinical trial when taken off choline enrichment but kept only on lithium worsened with regard to their manic depression.[15]

Lecithin seems preferable in these uses to that of choline. Choline must be administered four times a day at levels of 2½ to 3 grams per administration to keep the blood levels in the therapeutic range, whereas lecithin is like a time-released choline and only needs to be administered twice daily.

It is important to point out, however, that the use of lecithin and success with it is dependent upon the quality of the lecithin as it relates to its phosphatidylcholine content. For therapeutic success to result, the lecithin must be at least 30 percent phosphatidylcholine, with the higher levels having even more clinical success.[16] Many commercially available lecithins do not have this degree of concentration of phosphatidylcholine and are heavily diluted with other oils, and therefore will not be clinically useful.

Lecithin has also been found useful in improving acetylcholine levels in the peripheral nervous system and may help in thyroid-and adrenal-related hypertension (or elevated blood pressure) problems.

LECITHIN AND SERUM CHOLESTEROL

Clinical trials recently have failed to confirm that lecithin is useful in improving HDL levels or reducing blood cholesterol.[17] However, the emulsifying factors of lecithin help to make cholesterol more soluble and thus to prevent cholesterol gallstones. Other dietary variables which influence the composition of bile include copper, vitamin B12, folic acid and the amino acid methionine, as well as vitamin C.

In conclusion, it can be seen that choline and lecithin, preferably lecithin, can be used therapeutically, particularly in certain neurological disorders characterized by insufficient acetylcholine synthesis in the neurons of the brain and have found usefulness in the treatment of memory loss in the elderly, tardive dyskinesia and Alzheimer's disease-like symptoms, as well as peripheral nervous system improvement, particularly those connected to thyroid- and adrenal-related high blood pressure problems.

III INOSITOL

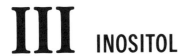

DIETARY SOURCES

The accessory food factor inositol is found in plants as inositol phosphate, sometimes called phytate. This material serves as a source of phosphorus in the plant during the germination process. The germination of a seed or grain will cause phosphatase enzymes to chemically cleave the phosphate groups off phytate, liberating inositol.

Inositol can be manufactured within the human body as well as in plant products, but again, its level of manufacture in certain individuals may not be optimal for their health. The dietary requirement in humans is still uncertain, and it is known that the synthesis occurs in the liver and by bacteria in the intestinal tract. There have been deficiencies identified in some tissues, and these symptoms include irritability, insomnia, hyperexcitability and nervousness.[18]

Dietary sources of inositol generally occur as myo-inositol and seem to be essential for the survival and growth of every human cell type that has been examined to date. It is interesting that diets high in unsprouted seeds and grains, which are thereby rich in phytates, may prevent the proper absorption of many trace elements in the diet, since phytates very effectively bind, or chelate the minerals in the diet, rendering them less absorbable. Either leavening of the grains or germination prior to their use will eliminate the phytates, liberating only inositol into the final food product.

PHYSIOLOGICAL FUNCTION OF INOSITOL

Inositol is another member of the lipotrophic vitamin family of nutrients which prevents fatty liver infiltration and works along with folic acid, vitamin B12, vitamin B6, choline and betaine, and the amino acid methionine in stimulating proper liver management of fats.[19]

Antibiotics which lead to sterilization of the intestine prevent inositol synthesis and may induce a deficiency symptom. Lactation without adequate inositol in the diet can cause reduction in body inositol stores and lead to fatty liver syndrome in the baby even if the mother is on a low fat diet.

Clinically, it has been found that individuals on a low inositol diet have a reduction in high density lipoprotein cholesterol (HDL) but not low density lipoprotein cholesterol (LDL). The reduction in HDL levels may indicate increased risk of coronary heart disease; HDL appears to be a protective form of cholesterol to atherosclerotic disease.[20]

Inositol has recently been found to function as a cell growth factor, since it stimulates the manufacture in the body of complex phospholipids, or a class of fats used in the body for the manufacture of myelinated nerve material. Inappropriately low amounts of inositol can reduce nerve growth and regeneration.

The most important clinical manifestation of this observation is the recent work which has indicated that peripheral neurological complications of diabetes which involve pain in the hands and feet, tingling sensation, and numbness of the fingers and toes with reduced nerve conduction velocity can be treated by administering large therapeutic doses of inositol as a supplement.[21] This condition of peripheral neuritis is responsive to myo-inositol supplementation at levels of 1000 to 3000 mg per day. The average American 2500 kilocalorie diet contains 900 mg of inositol, and most individuals claim that this amount is more than adequate to meet the daily needs. In diabetics with peripheral neuritis, the level of inositol in the average diet is not high enough to be in the effective therapy range. When there is an increase from 770 to 1640 mg per day of inositol, there has been found a significant improvement in the sensory neurons of diabetics with neuropathy. The level of 1600 mg can be achieved by careful selection of certain foods for the diet, but in general it is very difficult to achieve from dietary sources alone and an inositol supplement may be required.[22] Table I outlines the foods highest in inositol with the corresponding amounts given per 100 gram edible portion of the foods.

Salaway in a clinical trial used 1000 mg per day of inositol as a tablet in diabetics to increase action potentials of nerves and nerve conduction velocity and has successfully managed peripheral neuropathy in many diabetics using this method.[22]

THERAPEUTIC USE OF INOSITOL IN HEALTH PROMOTION

Inositol is one of those important therapeutic nutritional agents which will find significant application in the management of neuropathy, particularly associated with diabetes and the attendant pain that occurs as a result of demyelinating conditions of the nerves. This demyelinization is similar to an electrical wire losing its insulation and starting to short out. The stimulation of the synthesis of the proper nervous system material occurs with therapeutic doses of inositol between 1000 and 3000 mg of inositol per day, some of which may be derived from a diet higher in beans, oranges, cantaloupes, grapefruit or whole wheat, and the balance by way of a supplemental dose.

IV BETA-CAROTENE

For some time now, people have been aware that vitamin A has been suggested to be important in reducing risk of cancer. This belief has led many people to supplemental doses of vitamin A. Vitamin A is derived only from animal products. Vegetable products contain pro-vitamin A, which is called carotene. Carotene is a plant pigment found particularly in yellow and orange vegetables, but also found in many green leafy vegetables, and is converted in the body from the carotene form to vitamin A in the intestines and liver.

One of the most important differences between vitamin A and carotene is that vitamin A in excessive quantities can be concentrated in the liver and other tissues and produce cellular toxicity, whereas carotene has not been indicated to produce any direct toxicity. The only side effects of high carotene intake are the yellowing of the hands, face and skin from its accumulation and a recent report of lowered blood cell type called neutrophiles. The signs of vitamin A toxicity are hair loss, headaches, dryness of the mucous membranes, and liver changes; carotene has not been shown to produce any of these problems with high levels of intake.

Recently, exciting new evidence from medical research now indicates that the major protective agent against cancer may not be vitamin A itself, but rather is a pro-vitamin A, or carotene. A study conducted by medical researchers from the Rush Presbyterian St. Luke's Medical Center in Chicago, the Harvard Medical School, the School of Nursing at the University of Michigan and Northwestern University School of Medicine have all concluded that individuals who consume diets higher in beta-carotene were less likely to develop lung cancer than those individuals who eat foods low in beta-carotene. This observation was the result of nineteen years worth of medical records of male factory workers from a Western Electric plant, indicating that those men who ate more asparagus, green beans, beets, broccoli, cabbage, carrots, cauliflower and other green and yellow vegetables had lower incidences of cancer than those who did not consume these vegetable materials frequently.[23]

This observation that carotene-containing foods may be the actual cancer preventing agent rather than vitamin A itself confirms other research conclusions developed from studies in Norway, Japan, Great Britain and the United States. The original theory that beta-carotene may be an important cancer preventive agent was proposed by Dr. Richard Peto, of Britain's Imperial Cancer Research Fund, who indicated that beta-carotene was somehow very important in reducing the risk of cancer in men.

The Western Electric study, which followed dietary habits of nearly 2000 employees in the Chicago area and classified the workers according to their eating patterns, found that those food preferences, when related to medical histories, showed that thirty-three men developed lung cancer during the nineteen years covered by the study, with only two of those cases coming from men who ate diets high in beta-carotene containing foods, whereas fourteen cases were found in individuals who consumed low beta-carotene diets. There was not a correlation between the incidence of lung cancer and foods rich in vitamin A, but only with the level of beta-carotene in their diets.

Dr. Michael Sporn, of the National Cancer Institute, warns in an article in a recent issue of the *Nature* magazine the differences between beta-carotene and vitamin A.[24] Whereas vitamin A can be highly toxic if taken in large quantities, beta-carotene, as was mentioned, is not toxic, although it can cause temporary skin yellowing. Dr. Sporn goes on to point out, "People should not rush out and buy vitamin A in the hope of preventing cancer....Foods rich in beta-carotene may be much more important in reducing the risk of lung cancer."

Dr. Shekelle, chief author of the Western Electric study, has recently suggested that people should eat one or two helpings of carotene-rich foods each day. In all, about twenty studies have examined the relationship between beta-carotene and the incidence of cancer, not just lung cancer alone. In countries such as Japan where yellow-green vegetables are common, and in the Philippines where people consume significant quantities of dark green leafy vegetables, both foods rich in beta-carotene, there are proportionately very low levels of lung cancer as well as total cancer.

In a large study done in Norway Dr. Bjelke found that low

consumption of vegetables was predictive of a high rate of lung cancer, again confirming the importance of beta-carotene in cancer prevention.[25] As with any area of new information, there are some contradictions within the field; however, despite these limitations all studies come to the same conclusion: that the beta-carotene content of the diet seems to be important in the reduction of the risk of developing lung cancer, with none of the studies showing an opposite effect.

Experiments are now under way to try to learn the actual role of beta-carotene in the body and how it might curb the development of cancer. The actual level of beta-carotene taken in the diet with one to two helpings of green leafy or yellow-orange vegetables per day is equivalent to 5,000 to 20,000 International Units equivalent of pro-vitamin A, or beta-carotene. This can be derived directly from the diet or by supplementation with an appropriate beta-carotene concentrated supplement, usually derived from carrots.

It should be pointed out that beta-carotene is not a vaccine against cancer, but it is just one of the many agents that may be helpful in optimizing the body's defense mechanism against the cancer-producing process.

Dr. Shekelle goes on to point out, "The consistency of the evidence from diverse populations, the graded nature and time sequence of the association, the independence from cig-arette smoking, and the coherence with the evidence from animals all suggest that a diet relatively high in beta-carotene may reduce risk of lung cancer even among persons who have smoked cigarettes for many years." This observation is one of the most exciting conclusions drawn from the studies so far. Those smokers who consume beta-carotene enriched diets seem to have much lower lung cancer incidence, similar to that of nonsmokers, than smokers who did not consume beta-carotene enriched diets. This indicates the powerful protective effect that beta-carotene is able to elicit against the lung cancer production process, even in smokers. The research work at this point is optimistic as it relates to the important role that beta-carotene plays in promoting defense against cancer. The stage is set for the development and implementation of the higher beta-carotene enriched diet in the prevention of lung cancer.

Again, it should be recalled that beta-carotene is an accessory nutrient, certainly not suggested to be an essential vitamin factor. Its role in cancer prevention may be very different from that in sources of vitamin A, and it may not be considered to be a required substance for growth and development; but it may activate certain aspects of the immune function for optimal cancer prevention. Implementation of these new beta-carotene enriched diets will allow a more complete testing of the hypothesis that this substance is a powerful cancer preventive agent at dose equivalents between 5,000 and 50,000 International Units of carotene per day.

V   THE FUTURE DIRECTION AND USEFULNESS OF THE ACCESSORY NUTRIENT FAMILY

In this short monograph we have explored the clinical utility of four of the accessory food factors. This is just a small sampling of the total family of substances that are now known when concentrated from food to have clinical utility at therapeutic levels in specific individuals. It should be remembered that for one individual an accessory food factor may not be required because his or her body is capable of manufacturing adequate levels, whereas in another individual that factor may be an essential nutrient, either because of the metabolic inability to manufacture the substance or a specific disease process that may require augmented supplies to normalize function.

It is clear that not all individuals should be supplementing with accessory food factors, but that for those individuals who have specific metabolic or health requirements these agents when given therapeutically can prove extremely helpful in promoting health and proper function.

As we learn more about this exciting family of food concentrates and their implications on improving cellular function in specific individuals, the list of these agents will grow and become better established. The future is bright for this area of clinical nutrition but is one that will be continuously fraught with controversy, because these substances do not have a distinct deficiency symptom associated with their absence in the diet, but rather long-term evidence that their absence in adequate amounts may lead to chronic impairment of health. Most of our understanding of the essential nutrients is built around the concept that absence from the diet produces a deficiency disease, as the absence of vitamin C leading to scurvy and the absence of the B-complex vitamins leading to beri-beri or pellagra.

In the case of the accessory food factors, however, there is no acute deficiency disease which results from their absence because the body is able to manufacture some by its own processes. The challenge before the clinical nutritionist who is exploring the role and usefulness of members of the accessory food factor family is to identify those people who are at risk to deficiency of these agents and who have inherent need for supplementation of one or more of this family. The next five years should be most exciting in addressing these problems and more clearly defining where these substances have clinical utility.

REFERENCES

1. Fujimoto, A. and Bessman, S.P. 1978. *American Journal of Human Genetics* 30:51A.

2. Bessman, S.P. 1978. *Nutrition Reviews* 37:209-220.

3. Williams, R.J. and Deason, G. 1968. *Proceedings National Academy of Sciences* 57:1638-1642.

4. Horrobin, D.F. and Manku, M.S. 1980. *British Medical Journal* 280:1363-1366.

5. Culp, B.R., Lands, W.E.M. and Romson, J. 1980. *Prostaglandins* 20:1021-1031.

6. Zeisel, S.H. 1981. *Annual Reviews of Nutrition* 1:95-115.

7. Beams, A.J. 1946. *Journal American Medical Association* 130:190-196.

8. Zeisel, S.H., Growdon, J.H. and Wurtman, R.J. 1980. *Proceedings of National Academy of Sciences* 77:4417-4419.

9. Kapp, J., Mahaley, M.S. and Odom, G.L. 1970. *J. Neurosurgery* 32:468-472.

10. Rama Sastry, B.V. and Schmidt, D.E. 1976. *Biochemistry and Pharmacology* 25:425-431.

11. Jensen, R.G., Hagerty, M.M. and McMahon, K.E. 1978. *American Journal of Clinical Nutrition* 31:990-1016.

12. McGeer, P.L. and McGeer, E.G. 1979. *Nutrition and the Brain.* New York: Raven Press, pp. 141-176.

13. Davis, K.L., Berger, P.A. and Hollister, L.E. 1975. *New England Journal of Medicine* 293:152.

14. Boyd, W.D. and McQueen, J. 1977. *Lancet* 2:711.

15. Cohen, B.M., Miller, A.L. and Lipinski, J. 1980. *American Journal of Psyc atry* 137:242-243.

16. Steigmann, F., Finestein, R. and De La Huerga, J. 1952. *Federation Proce ings* 11:393.

17. ter Well, H.F., vanGent, C.M. and Dekker, W. 1974. *Acta Med. Scandinavian* 195:267-271.

18. Kuksis, A. and MooKerjea, S. 1978. *Nutrition Reviews* 36:233-237.

19. Gavin, G. and McHenry, E.W. 1941. *Journal Biological Chemistry* 139:485.

20. Ockner, R.K., Hughes, F.B. and Isselbacher, K.J. 1969. *Journal Clinical Investigation* 48:2367-2371.

21. Clements, R.S. and Darnell, B. 1980. *American Journal Clinical Nutrition* 33:1954-1967.

22. Salaway, J.G., Whitehead, L. and Payne, R.E. 1978. *Lancet* December 16, pp. 1282-1284.

23. Shekelle, A. 1981. *Lancet* pp. 1185-1189.

24. Sporn, M. 1980. *Nature* 136:582-584.

25. Bjelke, T. 1975. *International Journal of Cancer* 35:561-565.

FIGURE I
The Lecithin Molecule

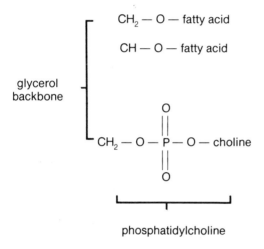

phosphatidylcholine

TABLE I

Myo-Inositol Content of Selected Foods[21]

Food	Serving	mg/serving
Pole beans	½ c.	175
Green beans, shelled	½ c.	193
Cantaloupe	¼	355
Orange, fresh	1	307
Grapefruit, fresh	½	199
Lime	1	194
Grapefruit juice	½ c.	456
Orange juice	½ c.	244
Whole wheat bread (stone ground)	1 slice	287
Beans, cooked	½ c.	283

KEATS GOOD HEALTH GUIDES

25 Titles in Print or Preparation...
$1.45 per copy
Editors: Richard A. Passwater, Ph.D. and
Earl Mindell, R.Ph., Ph.D.

- **Vitamin B3 (Niacin)** by Abram Hoffer, M.D., Ph.D.
- **GTF Chromium** by Richard A. Passwater, Ph.D.
- **Nutritional Parenting** by Sara Sloan
- **Tofu, Tempeh, Miso and Other Soyfoods** by Richard Leviton
- **A Stress Test for Children** by Jerome Vogel, M.D.
- **Choline, Lecithin, Inositol & Other "Accessory" Nutrients Vol. 1** by Jeffrey Bland, Ph.D
- **Octacosanol, Carnitine & Other "Accessory" Nutrients Vol. 2** by Jeffrey Bland, Ph.D.
- **Lysine, Tryptophan & Other Amino Acids** by Robert Garrison, Jr., R.Ph., M.A.
- **The Vitamin Robbers** by Earl Mindell, R.Ph., Ph.D.
- **A Nutritional Guide for the Problem Drinker** by Ruth Guenther, Ph.D.
- **A Nutritional Guide for Women's Problems** by Nikki Goldbeck
- **Nutrition and Exercise for the Over 50s** by Susan Smith Jones
- **Vitamin C Updated** by Jack Joseph Challem
- **First Aid With Herbs** by John Heinerman
- **Garlic** by Lloyd J. Harris
- **Vitamin E Updated** by Len Mervyn, Ph.D.
- **Hypoglycemia** by Marilyn Light
- **EPA — Marine Lipids** by Richard A. Passwater, Ph.D.